SQUARING THE CURVE

LIVING LONGER IN THE WELLNESS ZONE

Earl L. Kemper

authorHOUSE

AuthorHouse™
1663 Liberty Drive
Bloomington, IN 47403
www.authorhouse.com
Phone: 833-262-8899

Published by AuthorHouse 10/15/2024

ISBN: 979-8-8230-3220-9 (sc)
ISBN: 979-8-8230-3219-3 (hc)
ISBN: 979-8-8230-3221-6 (e)

Library of Congress Control Number: 2024921627

Print information available on the last page.

Any people depicted in stock imagery provided by Getty Images are models, and such images are being used for illustrative purposes only.
Certain stock imagery © Getty Images.

This book is printed on acid-free paper.

CONTENTS

ACKNOWLEDGMENTS

People seeking natural health freely share their insights and beliefs. Many of those people have influenced my beliefs and shaped my concepts about health during the last twenty-eight years. Specific individuals have made a lasting impact on me. I attempt here to recognize key individuals.

Clinton Howard, entrepreneur

- discovered that polysaccharides were the key ingredients of aloe vera that imparted its health benefits
- introduced the concept of "squaring the curve"

Dr. Reginald McDaniel, MD

- helped formulate and promote a powdered form of polysaccharides
- revealed a critical role of polysaccharides in cell-to-cell communication, thereby improving the effectiveness of the immune system
- explained why polysaccharides are lacking in our food supply

Dr. Alex Omelchuk, MD

- shared how he completely recovered from the debilitating effects of a hemorrhagic stroke many years prior by taking polysaccharide supplements
- reiterated their role in cell-to-cell communication

Dr. Neil Riordan, PhD

- introduced a nutritional product that nurtures the body to produce and make available stem cells to repair damaged tissue

Ron Keller, medical physicist

- a researcher who studied cancer at a major hospital
- personally developed cancer and successfully recovered using nutritional supplements
- *Forbidden Medicine* book reveals the true story of Ron and his brother

Dr. Neecie Moore, PhD

- advocate of a healthy eating plan
- author of *What's a Nice Person Like Me Doing in a Body Like This?*

In addition, my thanks to many people who supported me during my journey, including, but certainly not limited to, JC and Karen Spencer, Joe Woolsey, Ron and Sandy Brittain, and Ron and Lois Zehr.

Finally, special thanks to my wife, Dottie, who shared the journey with me, supported me in my passion, and reviewed and edited all my work before it was ever published.

INTRODUCTION

This book is about wellness. What it is. How to maintain it. How to recover it if it is gone. It is written for those aspiring to wellness and seeking guidance on how to achieve it.

A common belief is that if you're not sick, you're healthy. Yet people who think they are healthy die from their first heart attack, suffer broken bones from stepping off a curb, and learn they have stage four lung cancer. Wellness is obviously something other than feeling healthy.

This book asserts that wellness is about cells that function properly. The body is comprised almost entirely of cells and connective tissues made by cells. Every cell in the body has a master plan for the roles it should perform and the tools to implement that plan. If every cell is functioning as designed, the body should be working perfectly. That seems to be the best description of wellness. Malfunctioning cells fail to carry out their roles. When enough cells malfunction, symptoms arise.

Why do some people stay healthy longer than others? Good genes are not the answer. A study of identical twins concluded that genes account for about 16 percent of health conditions. The remainder is attributable to the conditions to which the body is exposed.

You are responsible for the 84 percent that affects your health. Your doctors are not responsible. Your parents are not responsible. The government is not responsible. As the one responsible, shouldn't you learn how to make wise decisions?

I've been learning about the body since 1995. My concept of good health and how to achieve it evolved dramatically over the years. I believed that if I wasn't sick, I was healthy. I believed that my doctors knew how to keep me healthy. But as I began to delve deeper into how the body functioned, I began to understand that neither of those was true.

This is not a scientific book, although it incorporates knowledge about the body. Much of the scientific bases comes from studies of biology, cells, connective tissues, genes, and DNA. Studies of wellness are rare.

There are things that we know about the body. There are things we know we do not know. And there are things we do not know that we do not know. I believe there are far more things we do not know than we know.

The foundation of this book is based on what we know about the body. Values of this book are often insights into what we do not know. A general rule of thumb is to do things for the body that we know are good for the body and not do things that we know are bad.

Take Responsibility for Your Health

You are responsible for your health care. When faced with a health problem, how do you decide what to do? Many people delegate their health care decisions to their doctors. People typically rely heavily on the advice and direction of doctors for solutions to their health care issues. For acute sicknesses or a trauma situation, doctors are probably the best option.

But if the health care issues are chronic illnesses and disorders, the medical industry falls short of effective results. As a result, the nation is suffering a health crisis. The costs of medical treatment of chronic illnesses and disorders are draining the finances of the sick and the nation.

Unfortunately, consumers searching for alternative approaches to chronic health problems are bombarded with conflicting information and advice. Free online advice is abundant, but almost all online sources promote a product or service. Criticism can easily be found for every option. A small industry of naturopathic practitioners and functional doctors address the needs of the body, but their advice is delivered one-on-one for a fee.

Consumers facing health decisions can easily be confused:

- What can or should they do to treat specific chronic illnesses and disorders?
- What can or should they do to prolong good health, delay aging, or prevent chronic illnesses and disorders?

Obviously, many people are making health care decisions that are not meeting their health care needs. Why?

Part of the problem is widely held beliefs that doctors know how to treat all health problems.

Part of the problem is confusing and conflicting information and advice about alternatives to traditional medicine.

Part of the problem is the costs of alternatives, which usually are not covered by insurance.

Part of the problem is that the health care industry is focused on treating sicknesses, not on promoting long-term good health.

Who are the key players in the health care industry, and what roles do they play?

The Medical Industry

- Medical doctors earn money from treating sick people.
- The pharmaceutical industry makes money from selling drugs to sick people. All drugs are toxic, and when used long term, such as treating chronic disorders, they will lead to further

health problems. To be classified as a drug, a candidate drug must demonstrate that it will kill 50 percent of the test animals. Called the LD50, this is a requirement of the Food and Drug Administration (FDA). If it will kill test animals, the drug will also be harmful to humans. The role of the FDA is to ensure that the benefits of the drug outweigh the harmful effects. If the drug is approved, the LD50 is used to set the recommended dosages for humans.

- Hospitals make money from treating sick people.
- Medical equipment manufacturers make money from selling equipment to sick people.
- Medical testing laboratories make money from running tests prescribed by doctors.

Treating chronic illnesses and disorders has become a major income source for the industry, especially the pharmaceutical industry. The costs of treatment are a major part of the nation's economy and are straining the financial resources of individuals, such that it has become a national problem. Politicians are extending hope of relief by proposing to bureaucratize existing practices that are not working. Nationalizing the existing health care program would enrich the medical industry, especially pharmaceutical companies, without solving the problem.

None of the medical industry makes money from healthy people. They have no incentive to teach people how to maintain good health, nor are they trained in how to do it. Their profits would be lower if people were healthier.

The medical industry is part of the problem.

The Health Insurance Industry

The insurance industry profits from managing the monies they receive to cover health care costs. They benefit from increasing health care costs. Their profits would decline if health care costs declined. They refuse to cover alternative health care options designed to promote long-term good health.

The insurance industry is part of the problem.

The Food and Drug Administration (FDA)

The FDA is a major influence on our nation's health care strategy. Even though food is part of the FDA's realm of responsibility, the actions of the FDA are dominated by the medical/pharmaceutical industry. The nation's food supply and diet are substantially ignored as potential solutions to chronic illnesses and disorders.

The FDA and the pharmaceutical industry work hand in hand. They need each other. The pharmaceutical products need the approvals of the FDA, and the FDA benefits from a more robust pharmaceutical industry, so much so that the FDA imposes restrictions on nonregulated entities that compete with FDA-regulated entities. The FDA actively persecutes entities that claim to "cure" a disease, a claim that can only be made by pharmaceuticals, according to the FDA. They do that despite rising evidence that natural health practices are more effective than drugs in addressing chronic disorders.

The FDA is part of the problem.

State and Federal Governments

The health care industry is a prime candidate for disruptive technologies, but state and federal governments have enacted laws and regulations that protect the health care industry. These laws and regulations make it difficult and costly for state-certified health care practitioners to prescribe treatments that are not recognized as "standard of care." Disruptive technologies will have to come from outside the highly regulated medical industry.

State and federal regulations, and their aggressive enforcement of them, are part of the problem.

The Natural Foods / Nutritional Supplements Industry

These industries sell products that supply nutrients to the body. Nutritional supplements are not toxic. The industry is competitive, and the profit margins are relatively small. They are not government regulated, and they operate within the constraints of state and federal governments. Their sales depend primarily on individuals who seek the health benefits of the products offered by the industry.

This industry is a natural source for disruptive technologies to the medical industry, but the costs of dealing with, and even fighting, state and federal laws and regulations are prohibitive.

These industries are part of the solution, but individually, they do not have the resources to take on all the barriers.

Consumers

Consumers make health care decisions based on beliefs about health care, on the information and advice available to them, and on the costs of implementing their preferred choices.

To reiterate—three key issues will affect their decisions:

- their beliefs about health care
- the information provided to them
- the costs of their options

Severe problems are associated with all three issues. Most people wrongfully believe that the medical industry can effectively deal with their chronic health issues, and the information and advice typically provided to the individual consumer is highly biased toward the medical industry. Finally, the costs of options not covered by health insurance can be prohibitive.

Because individual consumers have the power to spend their money where they choose, the power to change the health care industry rests primarily on their choices. But the choices made by these consumers are affected by beliefs they hold and biased information they receive. To make wise decisions, consumers need a sound understanding of what it takes to properly maintain the body and access to reliable and sufficient information.

Consumers have no one source available that can educate, inform, and offer sound advice that will help them make intelligent health care decisions about their specific conditions.

The purpose of this book is to help individual consumers develop a framework for making decisions that will help them maintain their good health.

Basic Principles

The following principles lay a strong foundation for natural health concepts:

- The human body is designed to heal, repair, and renew itself.
- Health declines with age.
- Health depends on properly functioning cells.
- The human body is always changing.

The human body is designed to heal, repair, and renew itself for its entire life.

This claim has four important concepts:

- designed
- heal and repair

- renew
- entire life

The key word is *designed*. But for the body to function as designed, the cells must have adequate key nutrients and a supportive environment. There are conditions for which the body cannot heal or repair itself.

People count on the body's ability to recover from infections and injuries. The medical industry relies on it. Surgeons rely on the body's ability to heal from surgery, even of patients who are well into their nineties. Doctors prescribe drugs to relieve pain and discomfort until the body recovers. The medical industry refers to health problems that continue beyond drug therapy as chronic diseases or disorders and claims there are no cures for them.

The nation's health care costs are skyrocketing because of these chronic health problems. An average of 75 percent of all health care spending in the United States is for treating chronic health problems. More and more people are taking drugs every day for the rest of their lives to relieve the pain and discomfort. The first chronic problem for people typically appears between forty and fifty years old. Subsequently, a second one will arise. Then a third and fourth. Obviously, treating with drugs is not the solution, but that's the regimen of our medical industry, and it's driving our health care costs beyond our ability to pay. The medical industry has built a huge business on the concept of relieving symptoms.

But what about the concept of renewing the body?

The human body completely renews itself about every ten years. All new cells and all new connective tissue. If the new cells and connective tissue are defective, this process contributes to the development of chronic health problems. This will be addressed a few pages later.

Health declines with age.

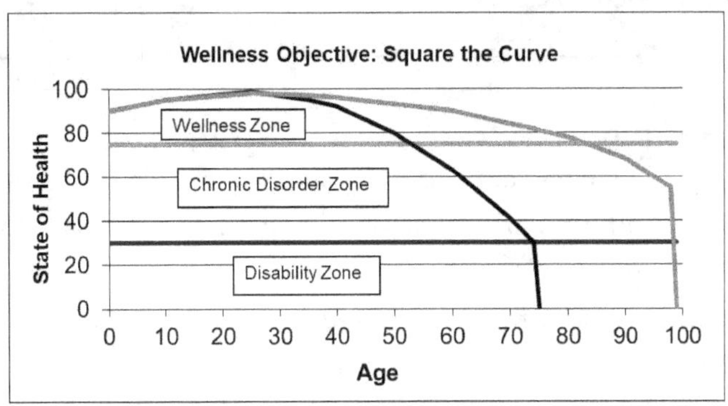

Figure 1. Health declines with age

Figure 1 depicts a declining state of health with age. Essentially, before death, everyone will pass through three health zones:

- a wellness zone in which the body will heal, repair, and renew itself
- a chronic disorder zone in which the body does not heal, repair, or renew itself, and the individual is taking one or more prescription drugs every day
- a disability zone in which the body needs assistance from equipment or other people

The objective of natural health is to prolong the time in the wellness zone and reduce the times in the other two zones—that is, delay the onset of chronic health problems. Chronic health problems reduce the quality of life.

State of health depends on properly functioning cells.

The body's functions depend on its cells performing their roles properly.

Chronic health problems are caused by cells failing to adequately carry out the roles they should perform. When too many cells malfunction, symptoms appear.

The body's state of wellness is directly linked to how well its cells carry out their intended roles.

- 33 percent—cells
- 62 percent—connective tissue
  - o 30 percent—loose and dense connective tissue (60–70 percent is collagen)
  - o 32 percent—specialized connective tissue
    - 15 percent—bones (30 percent is collagen)
    - interstitial fluids—12 percent
    - plasma—5 percent
- 2 percent—microbiome
- 3 percent—other fluids

Figure 2. Approximate body composition, weight percentage

Cells and connective tissue account for about 95 percent of body weight. Connective tissue, broadly defined, includes bones. These are approximate estimates because more specific data were not readily available. The key point is that cells and connective tissue make up the vast majority of the body.

The human body is always changing.

The human body is amazing! It is always changing. The body completely renews itself about every ten years. Cells and tissues are under attack by pathogens, free radicals, and toxins. They are damaged by normal wear and tear. And the body is working to repair damages to its cells and tissues, as illustrated in figure 3.

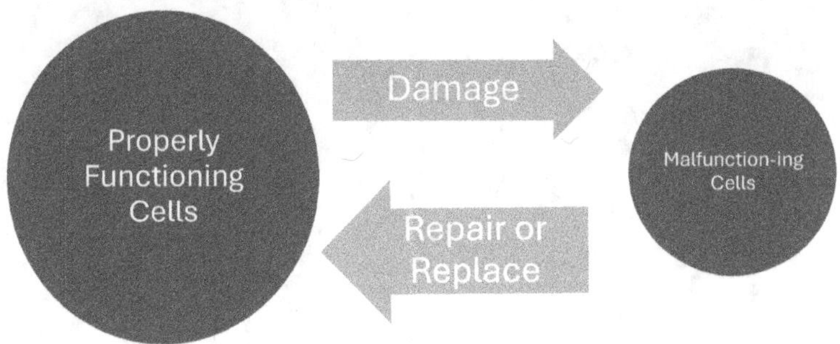

Figure 3. The body's cells are constantly under attack.

Properly functioning cells are vital for good health. Chapter 1 is devoted to cells.

CHAPTER 1

The body is comprised of a huge number of cells. Most estimates seem to be between thirty-seven and seventy-five trillion cells. Knowing the absolute number is not important. What is important is knowing how to keep those cells functioning properly, because the body's health is directly linked to how well its cells carry out their intended roles. Proper maintenance of the body's cells is key to good health.

More than two hundred different types of cells have been identified. Each of these types of cells has distinctive roles within the body. All of them working together with connective tissue carry out the functions of the body.

Stomach lining cells
Colon cells
Small intestine epithelia
Skin epidermal
Lymphocytes
Red blood
Macrophages
Endothelial cells
Pancreas cells
Bone cells
Stem cells

Figure 1-1. Each cell has dedicated roles.

Every cell exists as an individual, stand-alone unit, unconnected to other cells or to blood vessels. Essential nutrients needed by the cells permeate blood vessel walls and migrate to the cells through a fluidic connective tissue,

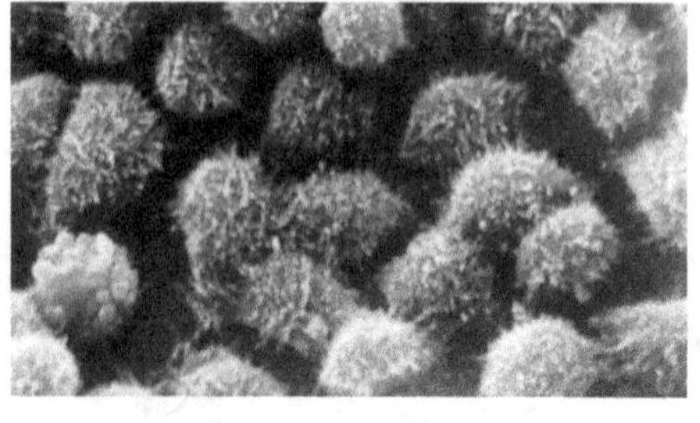

sometimes called interstitial fluid, surrounding the cells. At the right is a photomicrograph of a group of cells.

Library of Instructions

The roles of each of the cells are defined by the genetic code. The genetic code is a library of instructions for how to build the human body. The instructions are embodied within the 20,000 to 30,000 genes in the human genome. They make up the forty-six chromosomes, which may be thought of as separate volumes within a larger library, the DNA. Every cell contains two copies of the DNA.

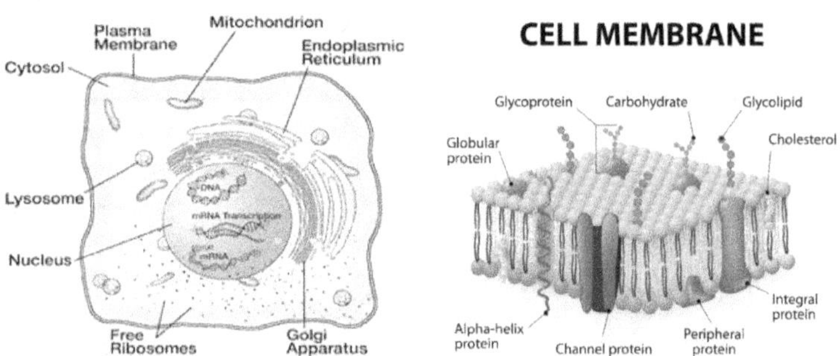

Figure 1-2

Components of a Cell

Figure 1-2 identifies components of a cell. The following four components deserve special attention:

Nucleus

    DNA—master plan for the body

    RNA—general contractor that implements the master plan

Mitochondrion

    Furnace—produces energy

Membrane

    Skin for the cell

    Receptor sites allow nutrients in

    Keeps out viruses/bacteria

    Cell-to-cell communication

Cytosol/Cytoplasm

    Raw/intermediate materials inventory

    Protein assembly mechanism

Each cell is contained within a protective cell wall (membrane).

Each cell contains a master plan of the body (DNA) that it follows to make its products.

Each cell contains a general contractor (RNA) that implements the specifications of the DNA.

Each cell has a site that produces energy (mitochondrion).

Each cell has a way to communicate with other cells (glycoprotein on cell membrane). (Glycoproteins are comprised of proteins and polysaccharides.)

Each cell maintains an inventory of the raw materials it needs (cytosol).

- The amount of nutrients stored within cells is significant.
- Cells account for about 33 percent of body weight.
- Stored nutrients may be 15 percent of body weight.
- A two-hundred-pound person would have thirty pounds of stored nutrients.
- The body does not store oxygen.

Roles of Cells

- A cell manufactures components of the body from raw materials.
- The raw materials (nutrients) are delivered to the cells via the body's delivery system.
- The raw materials enter the cell through specific portals in the cell membrane.
- The cell maintains an inventory of the raw materials it needs.
- Each cell is designed to produce specific products.
- Each cell has a site that produces energy (mitochondrion).
- Each cell produces waste products that are expelled through specific portals in the cell membrane.

Cells produce energy.

All the body's energy is produced by the mitochondria within cells. The usual process is to react oxygen and glucose, which produces waste products of carbon dioxide and water. But absent sufficient glucose, the mitochondria can generate energy from fat and protein.

The thyroid sets the amount of energy to be produced by the cells. A normal thyroid will keep the body's temperature near 98.6 degrees Fahrenheit. A lower body temperature can be a sign of hypothyroidism.

Cells make hormones.

Hormones are proteins, made by endocrine glands, that control many of the body's important processes.

There are ten endocrine glands, as illustrated in figure 1-3. Each of the glands makes one or more hormones. More than ninety hormones have been identified. Figure 1-4 shows what each gland monitors and some of the hormones made by them.

The thyroid gland controls the metabolism of the mitochondria. It determines the body's temperature and energy levels. The thyroid makes thyroxine and triiodothyronine.

The pancreas gland makes insulin, which is required to transfer glucose from the bloodstream to the cells, and glucagon, which converts fat from fat cells to glucose when needed.

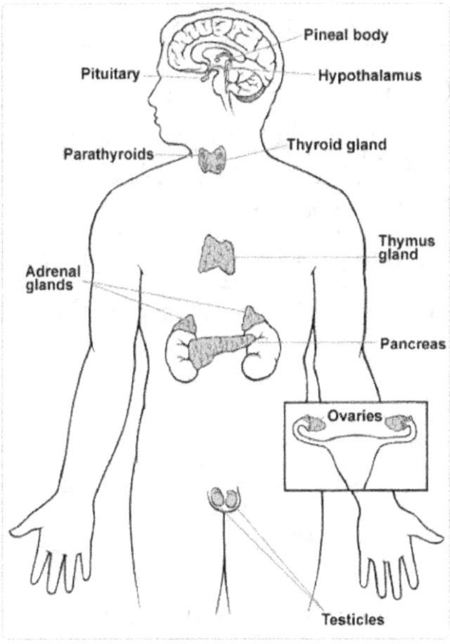

Figure 1-3. Endocrine glands

Gland	Monitors	Hormones
Pancreas	Blood glucose, proteins	Insulin, glucagon
Adrenal	Water, sodium, glucose	DHEA, adrenaline
Thyroid	Metabolism, blood calcium	Thyroxine, triiodothyronine
Parathyroid	Blood calcium (low)	Parathormone
Thymus	Immune system function	Thymosin
Pituitary	Other endocrine glands	Growth hormone, others
Hypothalamus	Adrenal gland functions	Adrenocorticotropic, others
Pineal	Daily physiologic cycles	Melatonin
Kidneys	Red blood cells	EPO
Gonads	Reproductive functions	Estrogen, testosterone

Figure 1-4. Endocrine glands and their hormones

Cells make enzymes.

Enzymes are tools the body uses to construct and deconstruct complex tissues.

There are three types: digestive enzymes, metabolic enzymes, and food enzymes. The body makes the first two. Food enzymes are contained in most foods. Food enzymes are why fruits and vegetables rot if not consumed.

Digestive enzymes help the gut break down foods that do not provide their own digestive enzymes into the basic nutrients that can be absorbed by the bloodstream. These foods typically are proteins and nuts. The pancreas makes enzymes that digest proteins.

Metabolic enzymes are the least known. Metabolic enzymes are involved in building complex tissues and breaking down waste tissue within the body.

I am profoundly amazed by the body's ability to build without flaw many complex molecules that involves coupling of amino acids thousands of times in the proper sequence. All the reactions are at atmospheric pressure and body temperatures. Scientists and engineers cannot do that outside the body. The DNA and genes provide the formulations, the RNA puts together the formulations provided by the DNA, and metabolic enzymes help connect the amino acids in the proper order and alignment.

We do not know how many metabolic enzymes the body has. There must be lots. An estimate I've seen is seventy-five thousand. To my way of thinking, there should be at least one type of metabolic enzyme for every potential pairing of basic nutrients.

In my opinion, providing the body with sufficient vitamins and minerals is key to effective metabolic enzymes.

Science has provided supporting evidence for this claim. Following are some known roles of vitamins and minerals in support of, or as a part of, the functions of metabolic enzymes:

- Vitamin C is involved in making collagen, elastin, and stress hormones and detoxifying heavy metals, especially mercury, lead, cadmium, and nickel.
- Magnesium is a cofactor in more than three hundred enzymatic reactions.
- Calcium activates various enzyme systems for muscle contractions, fat digestion, and protein metabolism, initiates muscle contractions, regulates normal heartbeat, and supports fluid transfer through cell walls.
- Vitamin D promotes absorption of calcium and phosphorus for bones and teeth.
- Vitamin B12 helps synthesize myelin; convert homocysteine to methionine; replicate the genetic code; the metabolism of folic

acid, proteins, fats, and carbohydrates; and the maturation of red blood cells, a critical growth factor for all cells.

- Folic acid is involved in synthesis of DNA and RNA, proper cell division, transfer of genetic code to new cells, healthy red and white blood cells, converting homocysteine to methionine.
- Iron is involved in oxygen transport by hemoglobin, metabolism of fatty acids, liver detoxification enzymes, enzymes that synthesize serotonin and dopamine, and synthesis of collagen and elastin.
- Copper is required for synthesis and function of hemoglobin and synthesis of collagen, elastin, and melanin (hair and skin color).
- Iodine supports the activity and function of the thyroid hormones.
- Selenium is a cofactor for glutathione and supports thyroid hormone production.
- Vitamin A is essential for all epithelial tissue, bone growth, soft tissue, and tooth enamel.
- Vitamin B1 (thiamin) has a major role in converting glucose into energy, maintaining nerve tissue, nerve function, nerve transmissions, muscular function (especially heart), and in the synthesis of fatty acids.
- Chromium increases the activity of insulin.

Thousands of chemical changes are happening constantly. All of them are most likely facilitated by metabolic enzymes.

Metabolic enzymes are essential for the body to heal, repair, and renew itself.

Cells make connective tissue.

Cells also make all the connective tissue, which accounts for over 60 percent of body weight. Because connective tissue is such a large portion of the body, chapter 2 is devoted to it.

Cells Need Specific Nutrients

Expressed as categories, these nutrients are as follows:

- amino acids (twenty essential amino acids)
- fats and oils (six essential fats and oils)
- certain carbohydrates (about twelve functional polysaccharides)
- vitamins (fifteen vitamins)
- minerals (sixty-five minerals)
- oxygen

These need to be supplied to the body. The body cannot make them. Except for oxygen, all these are supplied by way of our diet.

We maintain and replenish the cells' nutrient inventories through our foods and supplements.

If cells are deficient in one or more of the nutrients needed by the cells, the cells will be defective and will malfunction.

If cells are deficient in one or more of the nutrients needed by the components they produce, the components will be defective and will malfunction.

Defective cells may produce defective connective tissue.

Lifespan of Cells

All cells have a preprogrammed lifespan ranging from days to years. Figure 1-5 shows the lifespans of a few types of cells.

Days	Stomach lining cells (2)
	Colon cells (3–4)
	Small intestine epithelia (5–7)
Weeks	Skin epidermal (2–4)
Months	Lymphocytes (2–12)
	Red blood (4)
Months–Years	Macrophages
	Endothelial cells
Years	Pancreas cells (1+)
	Bone cells (25–30)

Figure 1-5. Cells have preprogrammed lifespans.

Making New Cells

The human body completely renews itself about every ten years—all new cells and all new connective tissue. If cells are not functioning properly, there is tremendous potential for malfunctioning cells to accumulate and lead to one or more chronic health problems.

Cells multiply by dividing.

The body is constantly making new cells. A reasonable estimate is one to four million new cells every second.

New cells are created by cells replicating themselves. Figure 1-6 is a photomicrograph of a dividing cell. To make properly functioning new cells and connective tissues, the mother cells need to function properly.

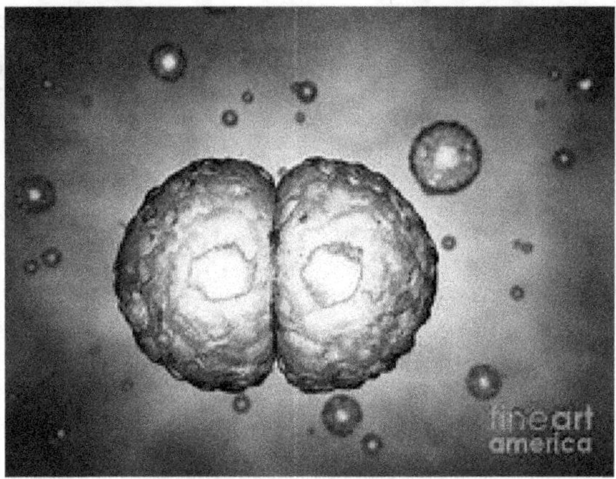

Figure 1-6. Dividing cell

To function properly, the mother cells must be supplied with specific and sufficient nutrients. Expressed as categories, these nutrients are as follows:

- amino acids
- fats
- oils
- certain carbohydrates
- vitamins
- minerals
- oxygen

These nutrients need to be supplied to the body. The body cannot make them. Except for oxygen, all these are supplied by way of our diet.

Without adequate nutrients, the mother cells will malfunction, and their daughter cells and the connective tissues they make will malfunction, eventually resulting in sickness.

An average cell replicates fifty times. If it is chronically malfunctioning, it makes fifty malfunctioning cells during its lifespan. As cells age, their performance also declines. Cells that have reached the end of their lifespan are called senescence cells.

Autophagy is a natural cellular process that breaks down waste products of aging or diseased cells and delays the aging process. Resveratrol and curcumin are believed to support the autophagy process.

Malfunctioning Cells

Cells working together with connective tissue carry out the roles of the body.

At any point in time, a portion of the body's cells will malfunction.

A healthy body will have a relatively small portion.

If too many cells malfunction, health problems will appear.

Sickness arises when too many cells are malfunctioning and the properly functioning cells are incapable of meeting the demands of the body.

The type of sickness will depend on the type of cells that are malfunctioning and what they are doing incorrectly or not doing at all.

The body's ability to heal, repair, and renew itself depends heavily on the body's cells properly performing the functions for which they are intended.

Consider the shingles on the roof of a house. Think of the shingles as cells protecting the interior of the house from rain, hail, snow, wind, leaves, tree limbs, squirrels, rodents, raccoons, and others. Some of the shingles can be damaged, and the roof will still be effective. But at some point, when too many shingles are damaged, leaks will appear. And if the leaks are too bad, the house will suffer internal damage.

Consider all the other components of a house—walls, doors, windows, furnace, thermostats, water pipes, sewage system, drains, showers, sinks, stove, pantry, floors. Any of those malfunctioning will create a problem.

In a way, your body is like the house. Your body has many different types of cells, each designed to carry out one or more functions supporting the body. If too many cells are malfunctioning, symptoms will appear.

Wellness is having properly functioning cells. And sickness occurs when too many cells of a specific type are malfunctioning.

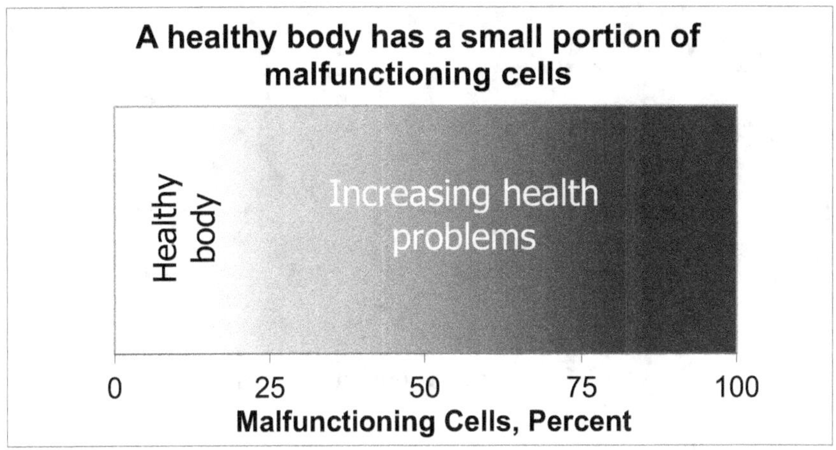

Figure 1-7

Causes of Malfunctioning Cells

There are essentially six basic reasons for cells to malfunction:

- pathogens
- free radicals
- toxins
- nutritional deficiencies
- overactive immune system
- acidic body core

Although the body is designed to heal, repair, and renew itself, to do so, it must be provided with all the essential nutrients that it needs. The last three of the above causes (nutritional deficiencies, overactive immune system, acidic body core) are all associated with a failure to deliver one or more essential nutrients to cells of the body, leading to cellular and connective tissue malfunctions that the immune system cannot correct and for which doctors have no cure.

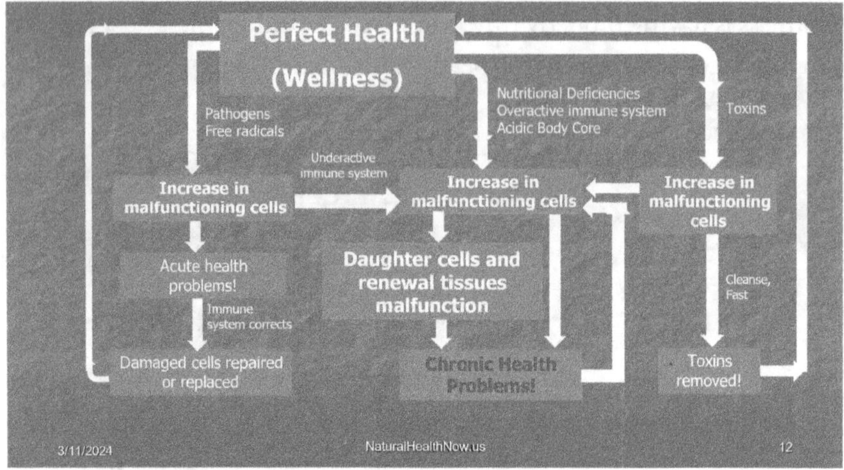

Figure 1-8. Causes of malfunctioning cells

Figure 1-8 illustrates the impacts of the six causes for cells to malfunction.

Pathogens and free radicals tend to cause localized problems. The damages they cause can be handled with an effective immune system and cells that were affected by them restored to normal functions. Drugs that relieve symptoms will give the impression of curing.

Toxins affect only those cells they contact. Helping the body get rid of the toxins via fasting or cleansing will restore the cells to their normal functions.

Key causes of chronic health problems.

Nutritional deficiencies, overactive immune systems, and acidic body core lead to malfunctioning cells that are widespread. The immune system is not designed to address these causes. If the causes are not addressed, the malfunctioning cells will multiply, creating new cells that will also malfunction, and the share of malfunctioning cells will continue to grow as cells multiply.

CHAPTER 2

Body Composition

Connective tissue is the most common component of the body. The table below presents an approximate estimate of the body's composition.

Approximate Body Composition, Weight Percentage

- 33 percent—cells
- 62 percent—connective tissue
  - o   30 percent—loose and dense connective tissue (60–70 percent is collagen)
  - o   32 percent—specialized connective tissue
    - 15 percent—bones (30 percent is collagen)
    - interstitial fluids—12 percent
    - plasma—5 percent
- 2 percent—microbiome
- 3 percent—other fluids

Cells and connective tissue account for about 95 percent of body weight.

What Is Connective Tissue?

The body's cells are not connected to one another. They are distinct units that are essential for the body to perform its roles. They must work together with other cells to carry out their roles.

Connective tissues help the cells work collectively. They are …

- the medium through which nutrients migrate from the bloodstream to the cells and cellular waste migrates to the bloodstream and the lymph nodes (interstitial fluid)
- the framework that supports the body's organs and systems (bones)
- the medium that transports nutrients, immune system cells, cellular waste (blood)
- the cartilage that separates the body's joints
- the cartilage that comprises the nose and ears
- the ligaments and tendons

Some connective tissue contains cells that make more connective tissue. Connective tissues are the reason blood vessels can expand and contract with each heartbeat. Connective tissues are essential for bone strength. Connective tissues make joint cartilage tough. Effective connective tissues are essential for wellness.

In summary, connective tissue …

- supports and binds cells and other tissues in the body
- maintains the form and body of organs
- provides cohesion and internal support

The most common component of connective tissue is collagen, which accounts for about 30 percent of body protein. Since about 70 percent of body weight is protein, collagen accounts for about 20 percent of body weight.

Because collagen is so prevalent within the body, a summary description about it is provided below.

Collagen

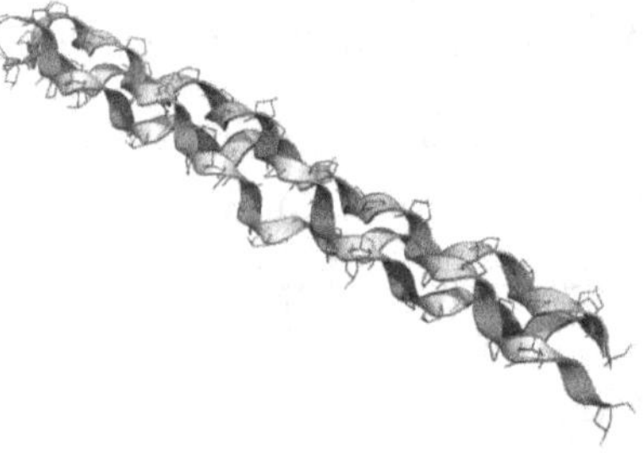

- Three helical chains of twenty essential amino acids. Each chain is about one thousand amino acid molecules long. Collagen molecules are too large to be absorbed by the skin. The gut breaks down collagen in the diet into smaller chains of peptides that can enter the bloodstream in the gut.

- There are twenty-nine types. The order of the amino acids within the chains will vary by type.
- It gives skin and blood vessels their strength and structure.
- It gives cartilage its toughness.

Primary Elements of Connective Tissue

Connective tissue is comprised of three primary elements:

- ground substance
- cells
- fibers

Ground Substance

Ground substance is a transparent fluid that suspends the fibers and cells. It has a viscosity of a watery gel. Its principal constituents are large carbohydrate molecules (polysaccharides), complexes of protein and carbohydrate (glycoproteins), and hyaluronic acid. Hyaluronic acid is comprised of glucuronic acid + N-acetyl glucosamine (a polysaccharide), chondroitin sulfate, and galactosamine (a polysaccharide).

Note that polysaccharides are important components of ground substance. A chronic deficiency of polysaccharides is common in the standard American diet and may be a cause of chronic health problems of connective tissue.

Cells

Some connective tissue cells migrate throughout the body (migrating cells), and some cells do not (stationary cells).

Stationary cells are fibroblast cells and adipose (fat) cells.

Fibroblast cells are the principal active cells of connective tissue. They make collagen and constituents of ground substance.

Adipose cells are the body's energy reserves. When we eat more food than the body needs, these cells convert excess glucose and excess fatty acids to lipids and store the fat for times when the body needs it.

Migrating cells are mast cells, eosinophil cells, plasma cells, and macrophages.

Mast cells produce histamine (affects vascular permeability) and heparin (delays or prevents blood clotting).

Eosinophil cells are a type of white blood cell.

Plasma cells produce antibody-secreting lymphocytes and immunoglobulins (antibodies).

Macrophages are cells that attack and destroy pathogens.

Fibers

Connective tissue fibers are classed as collagenous, elastic, and reticular.

Collagenous fibers …

- are made by fibroblast cells
- strengthen connective tissues
- are found primarily in tendons, ligaments, skin, corneas, cartilage, bone, blood vessels, and spinal discs

Elastic fibers …

- are comprised of elastin and are made by elastogenic cells

- give connective tissue elasticity
- are commonly found in arteries and lungs

Reticular fibers …

- are made by reticular cells
- join connective tissues to other tissues
- are commonly found in the liver, bone marrow, and lymphatic organs

Types of Connective Tissue

Connective tissue is classified into three types—loose connective tissue, dense connective tissue, and specialized connective tissue.

Loose Connective Tissue

Loose connective tissue is the most common type among vertebrates. It is the most common medium for oxygen and nutrients to migrate to cells from capillaries. Its fiber content is relatively low. It typically provides support, flexibility, and strength for internal organs, blood vessels, lymph vessels, and nerves.

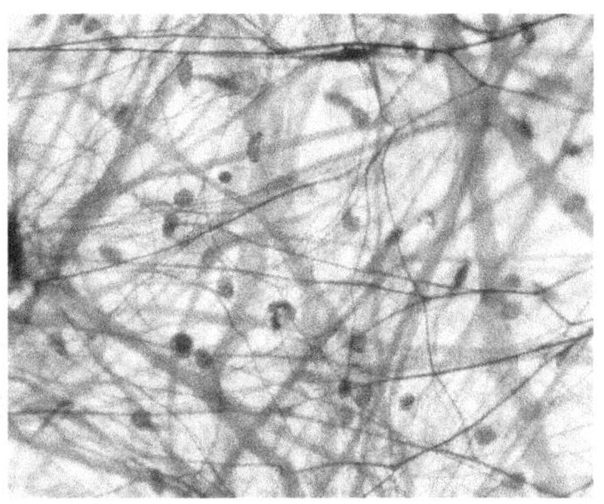

Dense Connective Tissue

Dense connective tissue has a relatively high fiber content. Regular dense tissue will be found in tendons and ligaments. Irregular dense tissue will be in

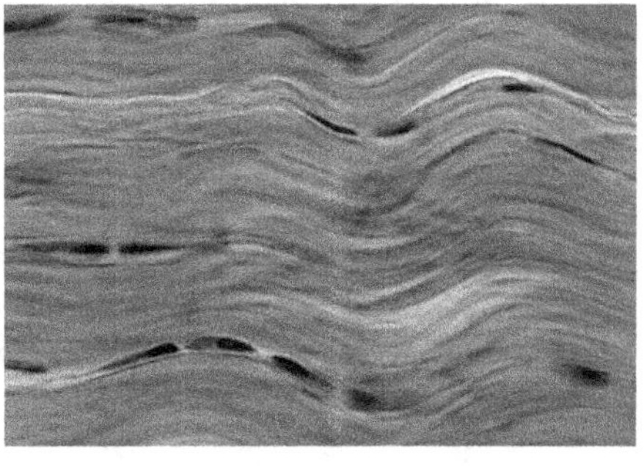

the dermis layer of skin and in membranes surrounding several organs. Elastic connective tissue will be in arteries, vocal cords, trachea, and the bronchial tubes of the lung.

Specialized Connective Tissue

Specialized connective tissues are adipose tissue, cartilage, bone tissue, blood and lymph fluids.

Adipose Tissue

Adipose tissue lines organs and body cavities, protecting organs and insulating against heat loss. It also stores fat in adipocyte cells and produces endocrine hormones involved in blood clotting, insulin sensitivity, and fat storage.

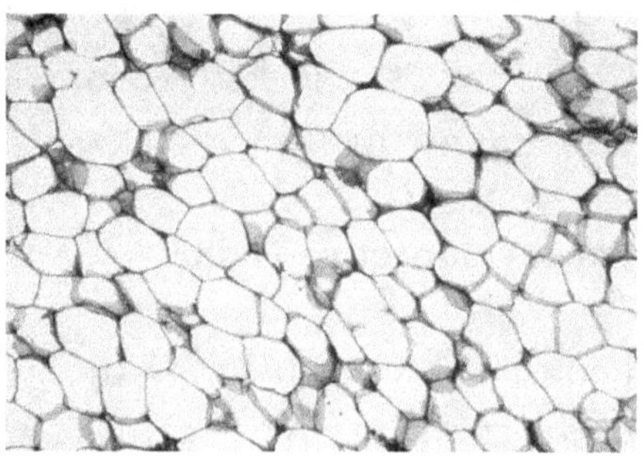

Cartilage

Cartilage exists as three types—hyaline cartilage, fibrocartilage, and elastic cartilage.

Hyaline cartilage is the most common. It is relatively flexible and elastic. Common applications are trachea, ribs, and nose.

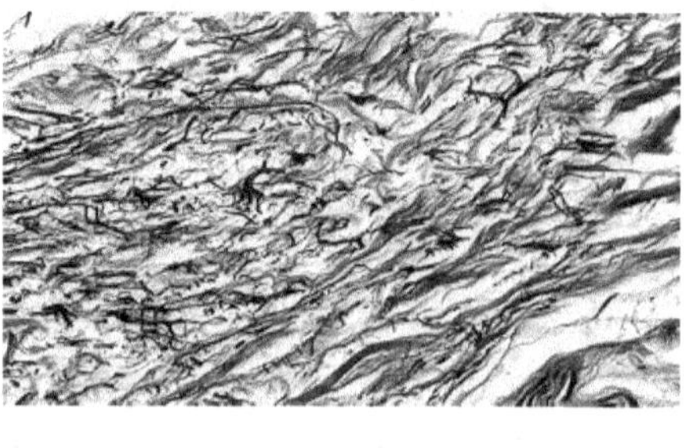

Fibrocartilage, made of hyaline and dense collagen fibers, is the strongest. Common applications are spinal discs, joints, and heart valves.

Elastic cartilage, the most flexible, is found in ears and larynx.

Bone Tissue

Bone tissue is mineralized connective tissue containing collagen and minerals.

Spongy bone tissue contains blood vessels and bone marrow. It is surrounded by compact bone tissue.

Compact bone tissue is a strong, dense outer surface of bone containing mature bone cells.

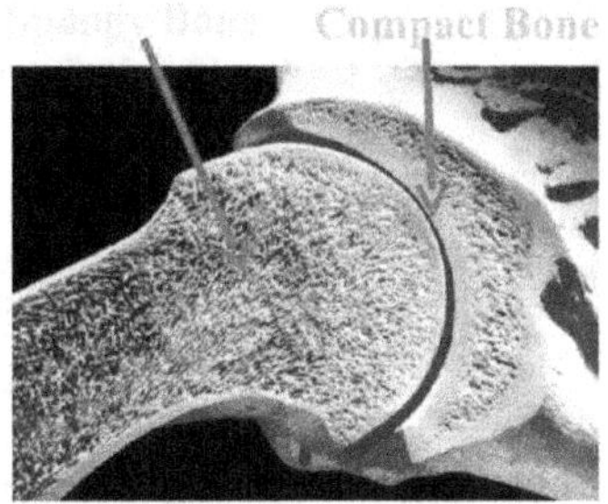

Common Health Problems of Connective Tissue

Connective tissues are made by cells. If a cell is malfunctioning, the connective tissue made by that cell may be defective. If the connective tissue is defective, it may be defective in its role within the body. If enough connective tissues are defective, the body may display symptoms. Connective tissue health problems can be caused by malfunctioning cells. Common connective tissue health problems follow:

- cardiovascular diseases and disorders
- osteoporosis/osteopenia
- osteoarthritis
- cancer
- lupus

Cardiovascular Diseases and Disorders

Possible Cause

> Plaque buildup on blood vessel walls is recognized as a major reason for elevated blood pressure and cardiovascular disorders. The body deposits plaque wherever tears appear in blood vessel walls.

What causes the tears? Each time the heart beats, the blood vessels expand. The blood vessels are comprised of cells and connective tissue. When the blood vessels expand, the connective tissue stretches. If the connective tissue is not strong enough, it tears.

Since blood vessel connective tissue is primarily collagenous fiber, weak tissue is probably caused by a deficiency of vitamin C, which is essential for making collagen.

Preventive Maintenance

Supplemental vitamin C.

Osteoporosis/Osteopenia

Possible Cause

The core of the body should be at a neutral pH of 7.0. The body tends to buffer excess acidity, but about the age of forty-five, its ability to neutralize excess acidity often becomes exhausted. Extracting minerals from the bones is a backup source of alkalinity.

Preventive Maintenance

Supplements that alkalinize the body core.

Osteoarthritis

Possible Cause

Osteoarthritis is bone-to-bone contact of joints due to deterioration of the cartilage between the joints.

The rate of regeneration of cartilage does not keep pace with the rate of destruction. Cartilage between joints is fibrocartilage, which is mostly collagen.

Probable cause is vitamin C deficiency.

Preventive Maintenance

Vitamin C supplementation.

Cancer

Possible Cause

The core of the body should be at a neutral pH of 7.0. The body tends to buffer excess acidity, but about the age of forty-five, its ability to neutralize excess acidity often becomes exhausted. As a result, the interstitial fluid of the body core gradually becomes acidic.

An acidic interstitial fluid inhibits the transfer of oxygen to the cells, depriving the cells of oxygen. In turn, the cells morph into cancer cells that can get oxygen from sugar.

Preventive Maintenance

Supplements that alkalinize the body core.

Lupus

Possible Cause

The immune system attacks the body's connective tissue.

A possible reason is the deficiency of polysaccharides causes fibroblast cells to produce off-spec ground substance that lacks one or more components of its normal composition.

Preventive Maintenance

Polysaccharide supplements.

CHAPTER 3

Signs of Trouble

When your car is acting strangely, you take it to a mechanic to find out why. The mechanic listens to the motor, takes the car for a test drive, runs some tests, and tells you what needs to be done.

When your body is acting strangely, what do you do?

This chapter is about interpreting signals from the body. It will not displace the services of a doctor. It is intended, instead, to help you understand the signals that the body is emitting. Sadly, the science relating the body's signals to causes is wholly inadequate. There are some books that address symptoms brought on by deficiencies of specific vitamins and minerals. Naturopathic doctors are trained in these skills. The purpose of this chapter is to address some of the signals.

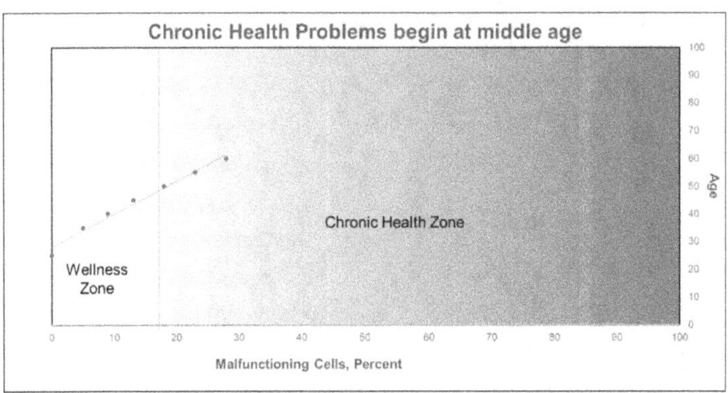

**Figure 3-1. Staying in the wellness zone
requires cell maintenance.**

When too many cells malfunction, the body begins to emit signals, commonly called symptoms. How to relate these signals to their causes is poorly understood.

At optimal conditions,

- the body will …
  - have energy
  - be mobile
  - be flexible
  - be pain-free
- the mind will be focused and alert
- joints will be flexible
- body fat will be low

These conditions may describe a body in the "wellness zone" of figure 3-1.

At suboptimal conditions, the body emits clues, such as the following, about what is wrong:

- elevated blood pressure
- high blood sugar
- joint pain
- chronic inflammation
- hunger
- sore muscles
- weak muscles
- cramps
- autoimmune disorders
- frequent infections
- moodiness
- low energy level
- skin sores
- wrinkled skin

- below normal body temperature
- brain fog
- chronic aches and pains
- chronic health problems
- acidic urine

Interpreting the Signals

These are my thoughts about the possible causes of specific signals from the body. I do not imply that any of the options will cure, mitigate, or prevent the symptoms for which the options were mentioned. Furthermore, I believe that many of the symptoms are caused by malfunctioning cells and that the symptoms will disappear if the cells begin to function properly. In this segment, I share my beliefs about what may be causing the cells to malfunction and what I would try if I had those symptoms.

Elevated Blood Pressure

Rising pressure in a pipeline with flowing fluid typically indicates that the fluid flow is being restricted. Usually, the problem is buildup of deposits on the wall of the pipe.

Elevated blood pressure suggests …

- plaque buildup within the blood vessels or
- reduced elasticity of the arteries

Both can be explained by connective tissue problems.

Plaque buildup may be caused by small tears in the blood vessels. The body fixes the tears by patching them with oxidized cholesterol—that is, plaque. The problem is that the connective tissue is too weak to withstand the stress of expansion each time the heart beats. Since collagen is the main component of the connective tissue, it is likely the culprit.

If the elasticity of the arteries is reduced, the arteries will resist expansion leading to higher pressure. Here again, the problem lies with the connective tissue, in this case with reduced elasticity of the collagen.

The body makes collagen. It accounts for about 20 percent of total body weight. To make collagen, vitamin C is necessary. Problems with collagen suggest a deficiency of vitamin C.

High Blood Sugar

Too much sugar in the bloodstream can lead to health problems. Glucose, an essential nutrient, is transferred into the bloodstream in the gut walls. As the glucose levels rise, the pancreas produces insulin and releases it into the bloodstream. Insulin is required to transfer glucose from the bloodstream to the cells and through the cell membrane receptor sites.

If the pancreas does not produce enough insulin, blood sugar levels will begin to rise. One cause of an underactive pancreas can be an overactive immune system that attacks the pancreas. An overactive immune system may be caused by a deficiency of polysaccharides.

Other conditions may cause elevated blood sugar levels. If the problem is not an underactive pancreas, certain supplements have proven to be effective at reducing blood sugar levels.

Joint Pain

Chronic joint pain is typically arthritis. There are two types of arthritis:

- rheumatoid arthritis
- osteoarthritis

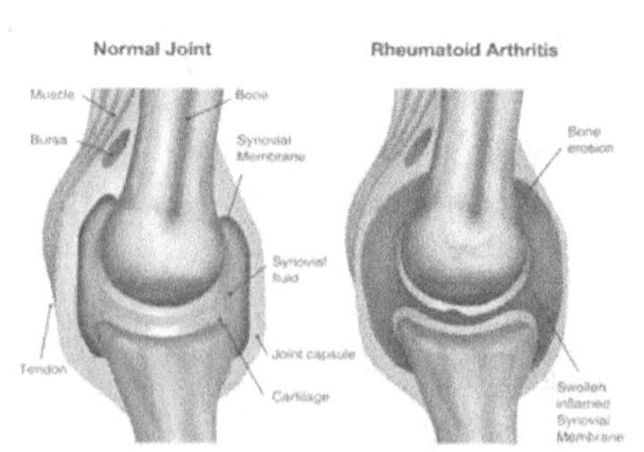

Doctors have no cure for either. They first prescribe a drug to relieve pain. Subsequently, they recommend joint replacement surgery.

The probable causes are different for the two.

Rheumatoid arthritis is an autoimmune disorder. The immune system attacks the joint leading to inflammation of the membrane surrounding the joint. The cause of autoimmune disorders is believed to be miscommunication between the immune system and the cells being affected.

The cause of miscommunication is believed to be a deficiency of polysaccharides.

Osteoarthritis describes the condition of a joint whose cartilage has worn down to where there is some bone-on-bone contact in the joint. I suspect that the problem is cartilage that lacks the toughness needed to prevent wear due to bone abrasion.

Collagen is the main component of cartilage. A deficiency of vitamin C can lead to weak collagen.

Chronic Inflammation

Inflammation is the body's response to tissue damage. The immune system is sending resources to the site of tissue damage to fight viruses and bad bacteria, repair damaged cells and tissue, and remove dead cells and tissue. All these resources cause the site to get warm and swell, or become inflamed.

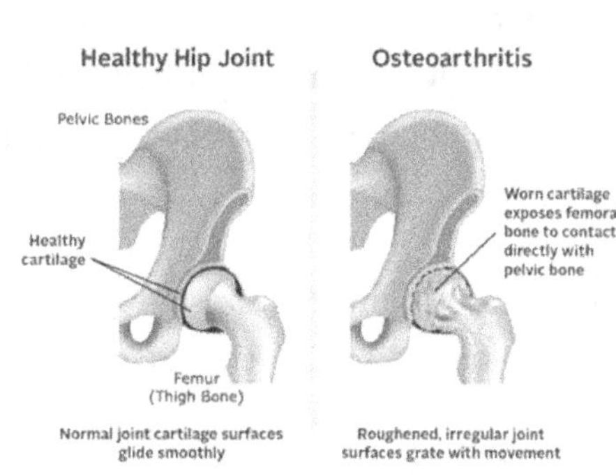

If the tissue damage is temporary, when the repair and cleanup is complete, those resources leave the area, and the swelling goes away. But when the tissue damage is chronic, when it happens frequently, that leads to chronic inflammation. Chronic inflammation can lead to chronic health problems wherever it occurs. In the cardiovascular system, it can appear as heart disease and high blood pressure. In the digestive system, in can appear as diarrhea, constipation, acid reflux, or inflammatory bowel disorder. In the lungs, it can appear as asthma or COPD. In the brain and nervous system, it can appear as anxiety, depression, or mood disorders.

Chronic inflammation may be caused by an overactive immune system, an indication of polysaccharide deficiencies. Other factors may cause chronic inflammation. Turmeric and curcumin have proven to be effective at reducing inflammation. Some formulated supplements containing turmeric and curcumin seem to be more effective than turmeric and curcumin alone.

Hunger

Hunger is the body's signal that it is missing a nutrient that it needs. Personally, I have not experienced hunger since I changed my diet in 2009 to focus on eating more raw vegetables, particularly complex carbohydrates, and very few high-glycemic foods. Even when fasting, I have not gotten hungry. I believe that is because I have provided my cells with enough of the nutrients they need to rebuild the nutrient inventories of my cells.

One type of hunger is caused by low blood sugar levels. Typically, this hunger appears several times a day, commonly every two to four hours. It is the result of low blood sugar levels caused by insulin spikes initiated by high-glycemic foods. High-glycemic foods spike blood sugar levels, which, in turn, lead to the pancreas overreleasing insulin. Too much insulin reduces glucose levels in the blood to below normal levels, causing the body to signal that it needs food. This type of hunger can be managed by changing the diet.

Another type of hunger is cravings. Most common are cravings for sweets and chocolate. Both are signals of a deficiency of polysaccharides, which are slightly sweet. Typically, if you supply the body with an adequate quantity of polysaccharides, the body's cravings for both will subside. Cravings for chips are the same, since chips are high glycemic and quickly elevate the sugar content of blood.

Sore and/or Weak Muscles

Muscles can be sore because of exercise or hard labor. That soreness is a buildup of lactic acid in the body. Lactic acid is the by-product of the body's process of destroying dead cells. Soreness from exercise or hard labor can be reduced by taking an alkalinizer to neutralize the lactic acid before or after workouts. By taking an alkalinizer before workout, you can exercise or work longer without soreness.

Sore and/or weak muscles can be caused by a deficiency of coenzyme Q10. CoQ10 is required by the mitochondria to produce energy. Sore muscles are a symptom of its deficiency. Taking statin drugs can cause a deficiency of CoQ10.

Cramps

Cramps can be caused by dehydration or a deficiency of minerals, especially calcium, potassium, or magnesium.

Frequent Infections

Frequent infections suggest an underactive immune system. Immune system problems are typically caused by ineffective cell-to-cell communication. Frequent infections indicate that the immune system is failing to quickly identify and respond to pathogens. Poor cell-to-cell communications are an indiction of a deficiency of polysaccharides.

Moodiness

Moodiness is commonly considered a hormonal problem. The body may be fluctuating between excess hormones and low hormones. Wild Mexican yam seems to modulate the hormone production—that is, it suppresses excess hormone production and nurtures more production when needed. There are several good formulated supplements that work better than wild Mexican yam by itself.

Low Energy

The mitochondria produce all the body's energy. Metabolism of the mitochondria is controlled by hormones produced by the thyroid. An underactive thyroid can be the reason for low energy. Reduced body temperatures are an indication of an underactive thyroid. Hormone production may be stimulated by taking iodine or hormone precursor supplements, but if the thyroid is already "dead," thyroid hormones may be required.

To produce energy, the mitochondria "burn" oxygen. Oxygen deficiency to the cells can also be a cause of low energy. Interstitial fluid that is too acidic will inhibit oxygen transfer from the bloodstream to the cells. Check acidity by testing the pH of the urine. An acceptable pH range is 6.5 to 7.5. Below 6.5 is too acidic. Above 7.5 is too alkaline. Excessive acidity is a common problem among people who are older than forty-five years. Adjusting the diet to include mostly green vegetables will help, as will taking "green" supplements and alkaline supplements.

Skin Problems

The skin is the body's largest organ. The condition of the skin reflects the health of the body.

Sores on the skin can either be from exposure to toxins from the environment or toxins inside the body. One of the ways for the body to deal with toxins is to expel them through the skin.

Wrinkles are often caused by a deficiency of collagen, the key component of connective tissue of the skin. Collagen is key to many connective tissues within the body. If collagen is deficient in the skin, it likely is deficient within the body. A deficiency of collagen can lead to any number of problems with connective tissue. Many health problems are tissue oriented.

Below Normal Body Temperature

The normal body temperature should be 98.6 degrees Fahrenheit. Lower temperatures are likely caused by an underactive thyroid. The thyroid controls the body's metabolism, which in turn establishes the body's temperature. If the thyroid is underactive, the body's "normal" temperature will be lower.

What causes the thyroid to be underactive? The common belief is that it is deficient in iodine, which is an important component of two hormones, produced by the thyroid, that control metabolism rates.

An iodine deficiency is probably not caused by a dietary deficiency but by the inability of iodine to get into thyroid cells. There are two possible explanations. Some evidence exists that fluorine, commonly added to municipal drinking water and toothpaste and offered as a treatment by dentists, interferes with the ability of thyroid cells to accept iodine. Another belief is that raw cruciferous vegetables contain a chemical that deadens the thyroid. Lightly steaming the vegetables destroys that chemical.

Chronic Aches and Pains / Chronic Health Problems

Chronic problems, whether they are simply aches and pains or are more severe, are almost certainly signs of one or more nutritional deficiencies. There are no tests that will identify the nutrients. Most naturopathic doctors will have ways that help them recommend supplements, but relating symptoms of chronic health problems to nutrient deficiencies is more of an art than a science.

As a rule of thumb, most people are deficient of polysaccharides, vitamin C, vitamin D3, and minerals. Polysaccharide deficiencies will lead to a malfunctioning immune system and certain connective tissue problems. Vitamin C deficiencies will lead to connective tissue problems. Vitamin D3 deficiencies will lead to bone density problems and numerous other issues. Mineral deficiencies will inhibit metabolic enzyme linkages in building the body's tissues. Minerals are cofactors in many metabolic enzyme reactions. Metabolic enzymes are essential in forming all parts of the body. Deficiencies can appear anywhere in the body.

Acidic Urine

The pH of urine is an indication of the pH of the interstitial fluids of the body core, which should be neutral or slightly alkaline. The interstitial fluids are the medium through which nutrients migrate from the bloodstream to the cells. If the interstitial fluids are acidic, they will hinder oxygen transfer, and the cells will be deficient of oxygen. Cells that are chronically deficient of oxygen will morph into cells that get oxygen from sugar. These are cancer cells.

Ideally, urine pH should be between 6.5 and 7.5. Below 6.5 is too acidic, and something needs to be taken to alkalinize the gut. A young body has the ability to buffer excess acidity, but that ability is depleted about age forty-five. The typical American diet will tend to acidify the body core. To offset the excess acidity, the body will begin to extract minerals from the bones, which will reduce bone density and bone strength.

Green vegetables are the basic foods that are alkaline. Almost everything else is acidic. The easiest way to neutralize excess body core acidity is to take alkaline supplements. Check your urine pH daily until you routinely get a pH of 6.5 to 7.5. The best time to check urine pH is right after arising in the morning.

Others

Other signals from the body are …

- cholesterol levels
- condition of stools
- sleep patterns
- condition of nails
- sense of taste and smell
- brain fog, memory
- hot flashes, night sweats
- headaches, migraines
- heartburn
- abdominal pains
- mouth sores
- overweight, underweight
- dark circles under eyes

These are all affected by nutritional patterns. Consult your sources of information for advice.

CHAPTER 4

ACHIEVING AND MAINTAINING WELLNESS

What Is Wellness?

Wellness is a state of health in which the body deals properly with its daily functions and with threats to its cells. It is not the absence of sickness. Pathogens (viruses and bad bacteria) may, on occasion, overwhelm the immune system for a short time. But the immune system of a healthy body will destroy the invading pathogens and repair or replace cells and tissues that were damaged.

Health Zones

Figure 4-1 illustrates that normal people will be healthy in their younger years, but their health will decline in their middle years and senior ages. The figure identifies three zones—wellness, chronic sickness, and disability. The objective of natural health is to prolong the time in the wellness zone and delay entry into the chronic sickness zone.

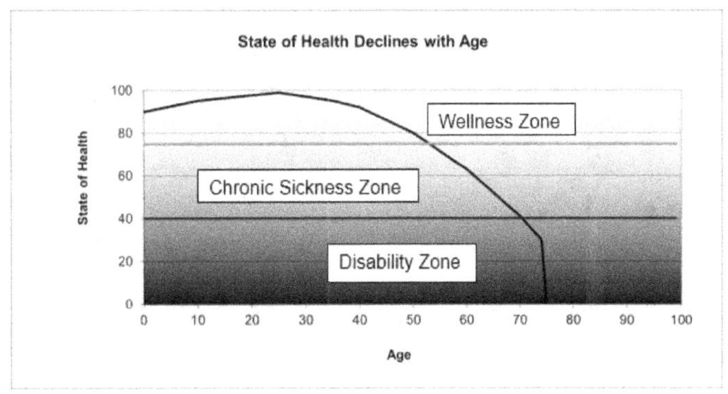

Figure 4-1

In the wellness zone, the vast majority of the body's cells will be functioning properly. Nevertheless, a small portion of its cells will be malfunctioning. Too many malfunctioning cells will lead to sickness. If the body cannot correct whatever causes the cells to malfunction, the sickness endures and becomes a chronic disease or disorder.

The body has more than two hundred types of cells. If too many cells of one of those types malfunction, the health problem that arises will be associated with the part of the body comprised of those cells.

Figure 4-2 relates the state of health to the percentage of malfunctioning cells. This is a hypothetical illustration. There is no known scientific evidence to corroborate the numbers, but it illustrates the importance of proper cell maintenance. Both figure 4-1 and figure 4-2 imply that entry into the chronic health zone for this illustration is at an age of fifty- to fifty-five years old.

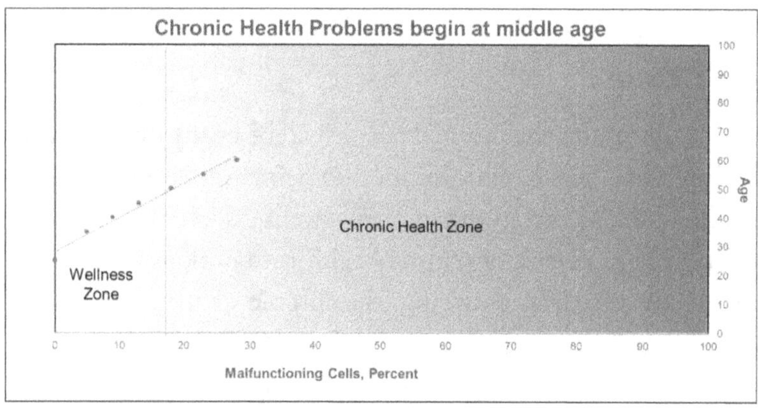

**Figure 4-2. Staying in the wellness zone
requires cell maintenance.**

Causes of Malfunctioning Cells

There are essentially six basic reasons for cells to malfunction:

- pathogens
- free radicals

- toxins
- nutritional deficiencies
- overactive immune system
- acidic body core

Although the body is designed to heal, repair, and renew itself, to do so, it must have all the essential nutrients that it needs. The last three of the above causes (nutritional deficiencies, overactive immune system, acidic body core) are all associated with failure to deliver one or more essential nutrients to cells of the body, leading to cellular and connective tissue malfunctions that the immune system cannot correct and for which doctors have no cure.

The buildup of malfunctioning cells in a normally healthy body is typically a slow process, taking years, as malfunctioning daughter cells and malfunctioning tissues gradually accumulate.

A normal baby is born with …

- all cells functioning properly
- every cell having a complete inventory of nutrients
- an innate immune system

The newborn has …

- no, or a tiny fraction of, malfunctioning cells
- hardly any antibodies

The baby's growth depletes the nutrient inventories of its cells. Those inventories must be replenished via its diet.

A normal baby has almost all cells functioning properly. A healthy mother's milk is filled with good nutrients for the baby, and baby food is nutrient rich.

As the child starts eating table food, the nutrient content of its diet tends to be deficient in one or more of the essential nutrients. That begins the depletion of the nutrient inventories of the cells.

Depending on the diet of the child, the cellular nutrient inventories gradually decline. Eventually, some nutrient inventories become depleted.

The cells with deficient nutrient inventories begin to malfunction. They make defective connective tissue and create malfunctioning daughter cells.

When enough cells are malfunctioning, symptoms appear.

All this may take thirty-five to fifty years. An adaptive immune system is built up by childhood diseases.

Immunizations help create antibodies. Are immunizations for children harmless? Many people contend otherwise, but that will not be addressed in this book.

The decline in properly functioning cells is likely due to *small* deficiencies of nutrients in the diet.

Those small deficiencies can be offset by nutritional supplements. It is wise to take such supplements while the body is still in the wellness zone.

Wellness Strategies

Every body has both properly functioning cells and malfunctioning cells. Both types multiply, creating clones of the mother cell. Malfunctioning cells cause damages.

The objectives of a wellness strategy are to keep the properly functioning cells functioning properly and to replace malfunctioning cells with properly functioning cells.

It is easier to maintain properly functioning cells than it is to replace malfunctioning cells and to correct the damages done by them.

Support Properly Functioning Cells

- Support maintenance and renewal.
- Suppress causes of malfunctioning cells.

Replace Malfunctioning Cells

- Support healing, repairing, and replacing malfunctioning cells.

Replacing malfunctioning cells with healthy cells is typically a slow process, taking months or years, as cell inventories of nutrients are rebuilt and new, healthy cells are created.

Most important are strategies to maintain the properly functioning cells, which are the largest portion of cells:

- Suppress possible causes of malfunctioning cells.
- Support the maintenance and renewal of properly functioning cells.

But it is also important to support the healing, repairing, and replacing, if necessary, of malfunctioning cells.

Key Causes of Chronic Disorders

Causes of chronic disorders can be summarized in three categories:

- nutritional deficiencies
- malfunctioning immune system
- acidic body core

Potential Nutritional Deficiencies

Nutritional deficiencies are almost always the cause of chronic disorders. A malfunctioning immune system is very likely caused by nutritional deficiencies. While an acidic body core may not be caused by nutritional deficiencies, it can be corrected with effective nutritional supplements.

Properly functioning cells depend on the availability of the following nutrients:

- twenty essential amino acids
- fifteen vitamins
- five or six bulk minerals
- sixty trace minerals
- six essential fats and oils
- eight to twelve functional polysaccharides
- oxygen

Provide the body with things that are good for the body and minimize the things that are bad.

These are things that we know are important:

- The body must be supplied with adequate amounts of essential nutrients to function as designed.
- The body needs favorable operating conditions to function as designed.
- Although the body has ways of handling toxins, the body can be overwhelmed by them.
- The body functions better with less exposure to toxins.
- All drugs are toxins.
- Most processed "foods" have additives that the body cannot use and treats as toxins.

We know a lot about the body, but there is much more we do not know.

These are some things for which we do not know the answers:

- How do cells make millions of long, complex proteins that are the same composition?
- If one of those proteins is not functioning as designed, how does the body know?
- If a protein has a bad molecule in its chain, can the body replace that molecule with a good one?
- How does the brain work?
- How do metabolic enzymes carry out their roles?
- What nutrients do the metabolic enzymes need to work correctly?

Dealing with Chronic Health Problems

Sicknesses and disorders are typically defined by the symptoms they generate. The medical industry focuses on the symptoms, and its protocols attempt to alleviate the symptoms. If they are successful, they claim a cure. If their protocols don't work, they declare there is no cure and label the sickness or disorder as chronic. For chronic problems, doctors prescribe drugs to relieve the pains and discomfort, for as long as the patient lives or is willing to take the drugs.

To solve a problem, it helps to know the cause or causes. Symptoms are evidence of malfunctioning cells. The dilemma is how to relate the symptoms of chronic health problems to the cells that are malfunctioning and whatever causes those cells to malfunction. So typically, we would try to determine the causes by reviewing the variety of symptoms.

The potential numbers and varieties of symptoms are countless! Each of the over two hundred different types of cells has specific roles. When these types of cells fail to perform all their roles, specific symptoms will appear. When enough cells fail in their common roles, the symptoms will be expressed by the body. Considering all the possible roles by these two hundred different types of cells, the potential number of symptoms could be endless.

The causes of the symptoms could be nutritional deficiencies, pathogens, free radicals, or toxins. Any one, or a combination of these, could be a cause. The following list illustrates the enormity of trying to relate symptoms to causes.

Potential Causes of Symptoms

Potential nutritional deficiencies

- twenty essential amino acids
- thirteen vitamins
- sixty-five minerals
- six essential fats and oils
- twelve functional polysaccharides
- oxygen

Others

- many pathogens
- many free radicals
- many toxins

If you have health problems, how do you identify the causes? Following are some suggestions.

A polysaccharide deficiency will lead to a malfunctioning immune system, which will lead to …

- autoimmune disorders
- frequent infections
- lingering infections

- allergies
- craving for sweets/chips

Vitamin C deficiency will lead to weak collagen, which will lead to …

- elevated blood pressure
- wrinkled skin
- sinus problems
- weak joint cartilage
- weak spinal cartilage

Vitamin D3 deficiency will impair calcium absorption, leading to reduced blood calcium levels, which may lead to …

- low bone density
- fatigue
- bone and muscle pain
- muscle weakness, cramps
- depression

A deficiency of minerals will lead to malfunctioning metabolic enzymes. which will lead to weak connective tissues …

- tissue-related health problems

An acidic body core will reduce oxygen content of interstitial fluid, which will lead to cells morphing to cells that get oxygen from sugar …

- acidic urine
- low energy levels
- cancer within the body core

The body's production of hormones declines every year after about age twenty-five, eventually leading to …

- reduced energy levels,

- mood swings, and
- hot flashes in women.

What Supplements?

Malfunctioning immune system

- polysaccharides

Weak connective tissues

- vitamin C

Acidic body core

- alkaline supplements

Hormone support

- hormone precursors

Generally deficient nutrients

- polysaccharides
- vitamin C
- vitamin D3
- omega-3 oils
- broad spectrum of vegetables

A malfunctioning immune system must be fixed!

A properly functioning immune system is *required* to heal, repair, or replace damaged cells!

Supplements to reduce inflammation

- turmeric/curcumin

Supplements to increase stem cell availability

- supplements that nurture stem cell production

Dealing with Aging

What is aging?

Aging embodies a wide range of changes that limit our normal body functions, make us more susceptible to diseases and disorders, and raise our risk of death. It's the accumulation of health problems that just won't go away—chronic health problems.

Signs of aging are chronic aches and pains, chronic skin problems, chronic low energy levels, and chronic disorders. The maximum heart rate gets slower.

Can the aging process be delayed? Yes. The solution is to minimize the causes of chronic health problems.

Chronological aging can affect the body's ability to heal, repair, and renew itself. Following is a list of known changes that occur with increasing age:

- Hormone production begins to decline each year about age twenty-five.
- Metabolic enzyme production begins to decline each year at about age twenty-five.
- Stem cell production begins to decline about age twenty-five.
- The ability to buffer excess acidity of the body core is depleted about age forty-five.
- Reduced ability to heal and repair leads to accumulated free radical damage.
- Slower cellular metabolism leads to reduced energy levels.

Most of these can be delayed several years with proper diet and nutritional supplementation.

- Hormone production can be nurtured with hormone precursors.
- Certain supplements can nurture the body to produce and release more stem cells.
- The depletion of buffering ability can lead to an acidic body core. A diet rich in green vegetables and alkaline supplements can offset a buildup of acidity.
- Free radical damage can be minimized by taking antioxidants.
- Cellular metabolism can be enhanced with proper diet and supplementation.

The table below indicates the age ranges for which health problems may arise from the effects of aging.

Age at Which Aging Effects May Lead to Health Problems						
Effect	20–29	30–39	40–49	50–59	60–69	70+
Hormone decline	x	x	x	x	x	x
Metabolic enzyme decline	x	x	x	x	x	x
Excess acidity			x	x	x	x
Stem cell decline			x	x	x	x
Free radical damage			x	x	x	x
Reduced energy					x	x

CHAPTER 5

The emphasis of this book is wellness. What it is. How to maintain it. How to recover it if it's gone. Maintaining wellness requires bearing the costs of nutritional supplements.

Most people at the age of thirty-five are still in the wellness zone without taking a nutritional supplement. Many people aged forty-five can say the same. Some who are fifty can also. Yet those are the ages when medical expenses begin to accrue. It's the time when most people transition from the wellness zone into the chronic health problems zone.

Some people will search for alternatives to drugs their doctors recommend. If they find a mentor they trust, they may start a nutritional supplement program. If it addresses the causes of their health problems, they will be satisfied with the results and continue taking the supplements for many years. An effective supplement program will delay medical expenses many years.

Figure 5-1 suggests that a wellness program may extend the time in the wellness zone by thirty years.

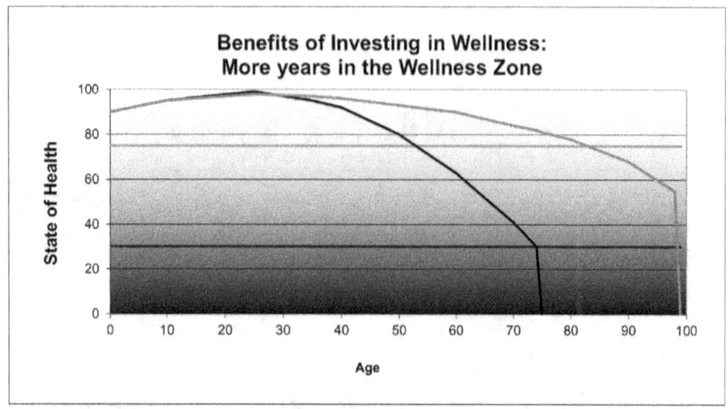

Figure 5-1

The Key to Wellness Is Properly Functioning Cells

The instructions for how to build the human body are embodied within the twenty to thirty thousand genes in the human genome. They make up the forty-six chromosomes, which may be thought of as separate volumes within a larger library, the DNA. Every cell contains an exact copy of the library. Every cell has the ability to implement the instructions for that cell, if it has the resources it needs and is in an environment that supports the cell.

All the more than two hundred types of cells have their specific instructions for their designed roles for the body. If they are deficient in one or more essential nutrients, they will not perform their roles without flaw. They will malfunction.

Wellness requires nearly every cell to carry out its roles flawlessly.

Wellness Program Options

How about starting a nutritional supplement program while the body is still in the wellness zone? How about early in the wellness zone when there are far fewer malfunctioning cells to cause problems? Maintaining cells that are properly functioning is far easier than trying to correct malfunctioning cells while at the same time maintaining the cells that are functioning properly.

Conceivably, there are two logical options for starting a wellness program:

1. Begin a wellness program when the body is at its wellness peak (about age twenty-five).
2. Begin a wellness program when the body is transitioning from the wellness zone to chronic health problem zone (about age fifty-five).

A wellness program started late will require more daily supplements than one started early, but the program started early would have the expenses of those extra years of taking supplements. This chapter looks at the costs of both options.

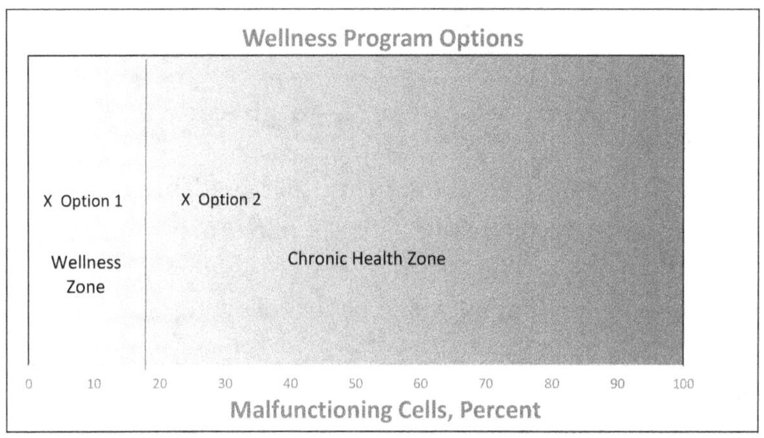

Figure 5-2

There are significant differences between the two options. Option 1 deals with far fewer malfunctioning cells than option 2. The primary objective of option 1 is to support and maintain cells that are functioning properly. Option 2 has two objectives. Option 2 strives to maintain cells that are functioning properly but also to correct cells that are malfunctioning. Option 2 is more complex. It requires more supplements.

Option 1: Begin supplements early in the wellness zone.

The objective of option 1 is to extend the body's time in the wellness zone by keeping the body's cells functioning properly. By starting a supplementation program when almost all cells are still functioning properly, the task of maintaining those cells is relatively easy.

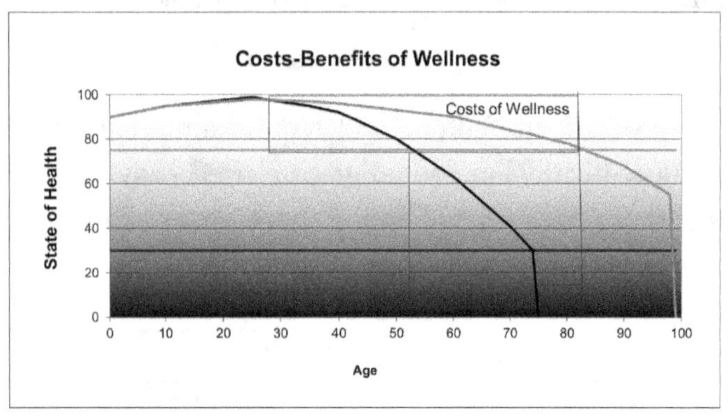

Figure 5-3. Option 1—Begin early.

An effective program provides nutrients that are deficient in the food supply and those that tend to be deficient in our diet.

A good supplement program would be the following:

Nutrient	*Start*
Polysaccharides	age twenty-eight
Broad spectrum greens	age twenty-eight
Vitamin C	age twenty-eight
Vitamin D3	age twenty-eight
Minerals	age twenty-eight
Hormone precursor	age thirty-five
Alkalinizer	age forty
Others	as needed

This analysis asserts that the costs of a wellness program are the total costs of supplements to keep the body in the wellness zone. Figure 5-3 illustrates the costs for option 1 which would cover the ages twenty-eight to eighty-two. The total cost estimate for option 1 is $295,000.

Option 2: Begin supplements after transitioning into chronic zone.

The objectives of option 2 are to restore the body back into the wellness zone and, once achieved, to extend the body's time in the wellness zone. By starting a supplementation program after chronic symptoms appear, the challenge is to correct cells that are malfunctioning while simultaneously supporting all other cells that continue to function properly. A reasonable basic program would be all the supplements of option 1 at double the daily amount. In addition, other supplements may be necessary to address symptoms that are problematic, such as high blood sugar, elevated blood pressure and overweight.

Option 2 raises the problem of an accumulation of malfunctioning cells large enough to create a health problem. It requires restoring the inventories of the missing nutrients in those cells and continuing to maintain that supplementation rate, every month for thirty years.

Figure 5-4 illustrates the costs of option 2 would cover ages fifty-two to eighty-two. The total cost estimate for option 2 is $320,000.

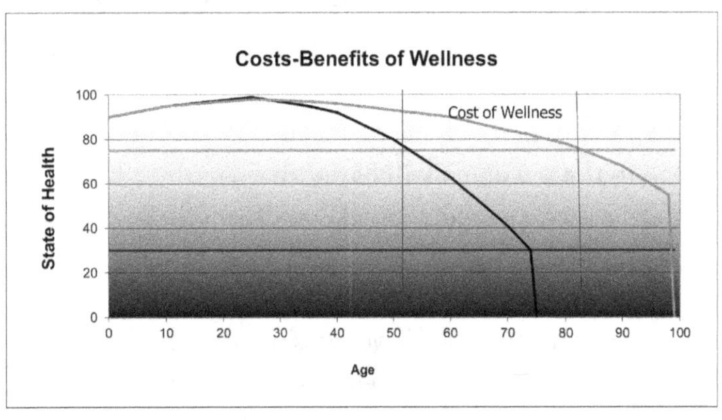

Figure 5-4. Option 2—Begin when chronic symptoms appear.

Figure 5-5 illustrates what the costs of each program could be. Note that these costs are only for supplements and do not include any other costs. In this illustration, the total supplement costs of option 1 are less than those of option 2 after age seventy-five.

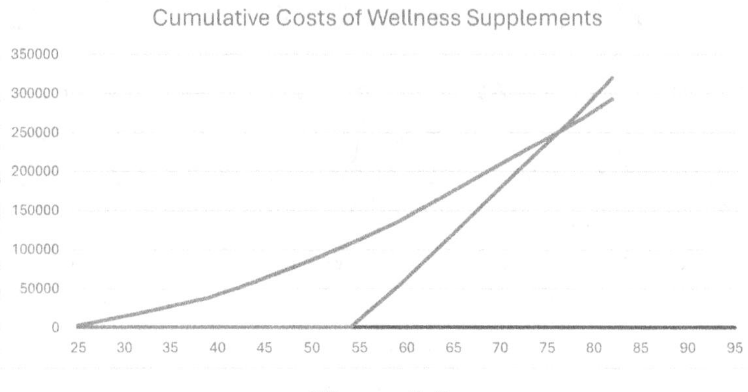

Figure 5-5

Health Care Becomes High Priority for Seniors

We are encouraged to save enough money to be able to do what we want in retirement. But most people who are in retirement wonder if they will outlive their savings.

For people in their senior years, health care becomes a high priority.

- Medical expenses increase 15–20 percent every year.
- Almost every senior over seventy will have at least one chronic health problem.
- One in two men will have cancer.
- One in three women will have cancer.
- One in two people over eighty-five will have dementia or Alzheimer's.

One of the potential benefits of a wellness program is significantly lower medical expenses throughout the senior years. Investing in wellness will result in more years in the wellness zone. The example in figure 5-6 illustrates an additional thirty years. The financial benefits of a wellness program are significantly lower health care expenses.

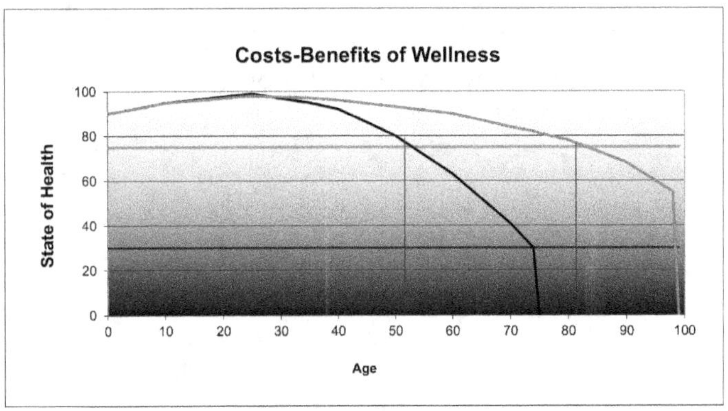

Figure 5-6

Benefits of Wellness

The benefits of wellness are both financial and quality of life. These include the following:

- o   minimal medical expenses
- o   annual physical only
- o   no daily drugs
- o   no office visits to the doctor
- physically fit
- mentally alert
- extended quality of life (thirty years)
- live longer
- independence
  - o   no visiting nurses
  - o   no home health care expenses
  - o   no assisted-living expenses
  - o   no memory care expenses

Potential Savings of Wellness

One of the benefits of wellness is lower health care costs. Following are estimates of potential health care expenses that may be accrued over a period of thirty years with chronic health problems:

Medical

- $1,000 per month for thirty years = $360,000

Hospital

- $10,000 per visit, ten visits = $100,000

Home health care

- $1,000 per month for fifteen years = $180,000

Assisted living

- $8,000 per month for five years = $480,000

Memory care

- $10,000 per month for one year = $120,000

Nursing home

- $10,000 per month for six months = $60,000

The total of the potential costs listed above is $1,300,000. Actual costs can easily exceed that.

Figure 5-7 illustrates these potential costs that could be considered "savings" for a person who maintains an extra thirty years in the wellness zone.

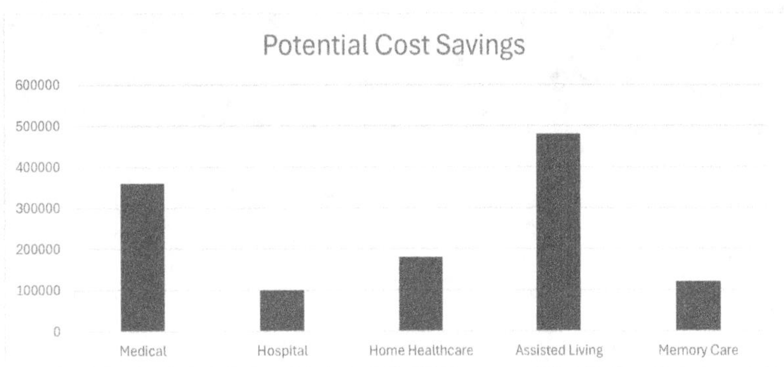

Figure 5-7

A good health insurance plan may cover most of the medical and hospital expenses totaling $460,000. Granted that, the potential costs not covered by insurance would be $840,000. That level of potential savings certainly justifies an investment of $320,000 for supplements.

Additional Benefits

Beyond potentially lower financial expenses, a wellness program delivers additional benefits. Here are the obvious ones:

- physically fit
- mentally alert
- extended quality of life
- longer life
- independence
- less stress (personally and on family)

Putting a dollar value on these is impossible. These alone justify the total costs of a long-term wellness program.

CHAPTER 6

FINAL THOUGHTS AND COMMENTS

This book is about wellness. It is not a book reporting the results of scientific research. It is intended for individuals who are searching for wisdom on how to make decisions that will affect their health.

The concepts in this book likely challenge the traditional beliefs of the reader. Maybe it's appropriate to end this book with some thoughts and comments that support these concepts. That's what this chapter is about.

What Is Wellness?

The best description of wellness is when all the body's cells are functioning properly.

If all cells are functioning properly …

- They will make properly functioning daughter cells.
- They will make connective tissue that functions properly.
- All organs and glands will function properly.
- They will make proteins according to their genetic code instructions.
- The immune system will be effective.

An effective immune system can deal with injuries, pathogens, free radicals, and toxins, if they do not overwhelm the body. We should not intentionally overexpose the body to these negative factors, but exposure will happen, and a body in the wellness zone can usually handle them.

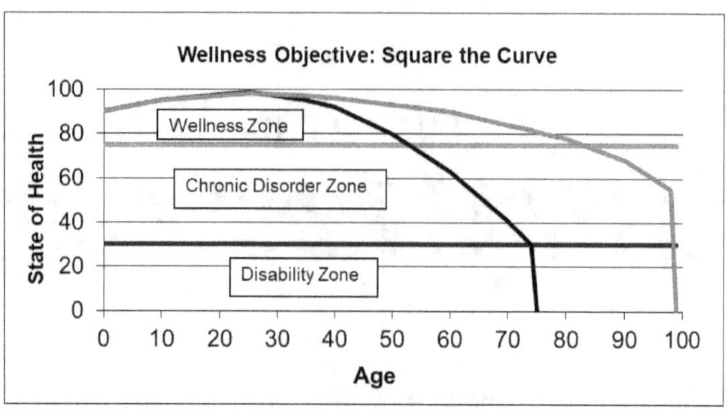

Figure 6-1

The concept of a wellness zone is illustrated in figure 6-1. When the body is in the wellness zone, it will heal, repair, and renew itself. When the body fails to heal and repair itself, given "enough time," it crosses into the chronic disorder zone. The traditional time frame for "enough time" has been three months, but some people are proposing that six months would be more realistic.

The black curve in figure 6-1 represents the typical path people today would incur if they did not make a specific effort to keep their body in the wellness zone. Note that the typical path stays in the wellness zone for about fifty years. The red curve in figure 6-1 implies that an effective wellness program can extend the time in the wellness zone by thirty years.

Why does a body operate in the wellness zone for fifty years or more and, thereafter, slip into the chronic disorder zone?

How can a person ensure that they are on the path of the red curve and not the black curve?

Beginning Life in the Wellness Zone

Perfect health is all the body's cells functioning properly. Properly functioning cells together with connective tissues carry out all the roles of the body. Cells make all connective tissue. When all the cells are functioning properly and the connective tissues are not defective, the body should be in perfect health.

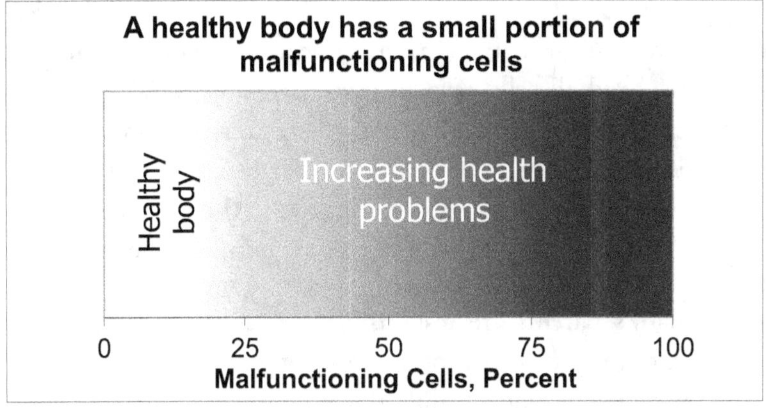

Figure 6-2

However, the body is designed to carry out its functions even when some of the cells are malfunctioning. It has more than enough cells to support the roles of the body even when some are not functioning properly. Figure 6-2 illustrates this concept.

If too many cells are malfunctioning, the body will emit signals. These are usually called symptoms. The medical industry focuses on these symptoms to determine from what disease or disorder the body is suffering. A common strategy of doctors is to prescribe a drug to relieve the symptoms until the body heals itself. When the body fails to heal itself, the problem is designated as a chronic problem.

How can a person stay in the wellness zone for fifty years without a wellness program? In the paragraphs below, I offer my unproven and unverified concepts. They are one possible explanation that is consistent with the concept of wellness basically being properly functioning cells.

A normal baby starts life in the wellness zone. Life begins as one cell with one sperm and one egg. The genetic code of that cell contains all the instructions needed to create a baby. The nourishment the developing baby needs comes from the mother's body. The baby's nourishment receives top priority from the mother's body, sometimes to the detriment of the health of the mother.

At birth, a normal baby is in perfect health. Every cell is functioning properly, and all cells have an inventory of essential nutrients. An abnormal baby may have a genetic defect that will affect its health. A study of identical twins revealed that heredity may account for 16 percent of an individual's health status. The reference here is to a typical baby. Obviously, some babies are born with health problems.

The baby's parents are responsible for replenishing the essential nutrients used by the cells of the growing person. And when the child becomes an independent adult, the responsibility shifts to him or her.

The transition from perfect health to the chronic disorder zone takes many years. The typical diet may be slightly deficient in one or more of the essential nutrients. Gradually, that deficiency will draw down and deplete the inventory of that nutrient, which, in turn, will lead to some cells making defective connective tissue and producing malfunctioning daughter cells. Over the years, the population of malfunctioning cells and defective tissue will accumulate and will eventually lead to chronic health problems.

Extending Life in the Wellness Zone

How can a person extend his life in the wellness zone? Staying in the wellness zone requires proper and routine support for the body's cells.

I'm convinced that what we do not know about the body far exceeds what we do know.

How should that affect our decision-making? A general rule of thumb is to give the body what we know is good for the body and to not expose the body to what we know is bad for the body.

Cells Need Essential Nutrients to Function Properly

To function properly, the body needs to have an adequate supply of essential nutrients. These are provided primarily by food, except oxygen, which our lungs extract from the air we breathe. What foods we supply the body is one of our most important roles.

Choosing nutrient-rich foods is preferable. Sadly, the nutrient content of the nation's food supply is deteriorating. And that is leading to a deficiency in the quality and quantity of essential nutrients provided to our bodies.

In addition, the standard American diet is rich in calories and lacking in essential nutrients. That, also, is leading to a deficiency in the quality and quantity of essential nutrients provided to our bodies.

When the body's cells are deficient in one or more of the essential nutrients they need to function properly, they malfunction. When enough cells malfunction, symptoms appear. This book contends that malfunctioning cells lead to sickness.

Because of the decline in the nutrient content of the food supply and the choice of foods by the typical person, almost all people are deficient in the following nutrients:

Polysaccharides

Polysaccharides are sugars that develop in fruits and vegetables in the last few days of ripening on the plant. Polysaccharides are why vine-ripened tomatoes taste sweeter than tomatoes picked green. Polysaccharides are key to cell-to-cell communication, which is required for the immune system to be effective. Polysaccharides are also an important component of connective tissues. Many fruits and vegetables are picked green, before the polysaccharides develop, so they can be shipped long distances. Green harvesting of fruits and vegetables has led to a deficiency of polysaccharides in fresh produce. A deficiency of polysaccharides may be the cause of autoimmune disorders, frequent and lingering infections, and allergies. It may also be a cause of health problems of the connective tissues.

Vitamin C

Vitamin C is required for the body to make collagen. Connective tissue is about two-thirds collagen. A deficiency of vitamin C may lead to the body making defective collagen, which may be a cause of connective tissue health problems.

Vitamin D3

Vitamin D3 is required for the body to build bones and teeth. A deficiency of vitamin D3 may be a cause of weak bones and teeth.

Trace minerals

Metabolic enzymes are key to the body's ongoing construction of complex proteins and other molecules. They unite two different molecules in the process of building proteins and other molecules. Performing their roles requires the presence of vitamins and minerals. Deficiencies of vitamins and minerals most likely lead to defective proteins and other molecules.

Basic nutrients

Plant-based foods are the richest in the nutrients needed by the body. Because our choice of diet may lead to a deficiency of key nutrients, a good strategy is to take a nutritional supplement that provides a broad spectrum of plant ingredients.

Cells Store Essential Nutrients

Since cells are constantly making new tissue, they are depleting essential nutrients from their inventories. Each cell maintains an inventory in the cytosol of the raw materials it needs.

- The amount of nutrients stored within cells is significant.

- Cells account for about 33 percent of body weight.
- Stored nutrients may be 15 percent of body weight.
- A two-hundred-pound person would have thirty pounds of stored nutrients.
- The body does not store oxygen.

These inventories are replenished when we consume foods and supplements. Since much of the food supplied by plants is seasonal, the body stocks up on those nutrients when they are in season so they are available when needed.

Interpreting the Body's Signals

When too many cells malfunction, the body begins to emit signals, commonly called symptoms. How to relate these signals to their causes is poorly understood.

At optimal conditions,

- the body will …
  - have energy
  - be mobile
  - be flexible
  - be pain-free
- the mind will be focused and alert
- joints will be flexible
- body fat will be low

These conditions may describe a body in the "wellness zone" of figure 6-2.

At suboptimal conditions, the body emits clues, such as the following, about what is wrong:

- elevated blood pressure
- high blood sugar

- joint pain
- chronic inflammation
- hunger
- sore muscles
- weak muscles
- cramps
- autoimmune disorders
- frequent infections
- moodiness
- low energy level
- skin sores
- wrinkled skin
- below normal body temperature
- brain fog
- chronic aches and pains
- chronic health problems
- acidic urine

These signals were addressed in chapter 3. This book contends that they are all the result of malfunctioning cells. The challenge is to discover how to address the causes.

Wellness Principles

Certain principles are key to wellness:

Ultimate wellness is when all the body's cells are functioning properly.

To function properly, cells need to be supplied with essential nutrients.

Cells that are deficient in essential nutrients will malfunction.

Sickness occurs when too many of the body's cells malfunction.

Chronic deficiency of one or more essential nutrients will lead to chronic health problems.

Keeping the body's cells supplied with adequate essential nutrients will prolong the state of wellness of the human body.

Closing Thoughts

A question posed in the introduction was, why are many people making health care decisions that do not meet their health care needs?

The following comments were offered in explanation:

Part of the problem is widely held beliefs that doctors know how to treat all health problems.

Part of the problem is an abundance of confusing and conflicting information and advice about alternatives to traditional medicine.

Part of the problem is that the health care industry is focused on treating sicknesses, not promoting long-term good health.

I believe that effective changes in the nation's health care will eventually come from actions taken by consumers of health care products and services.

This is my attempt to share with readers the factors I consider when facing decisions that affect my health. Some factors are concepts based on my assumptions and beliefs about how the body functions and are not based on scientific research. When a health problem is chronic, I will usually choose not to use drugs, and I may follow the advice of friends and relatives. If the problem is an infection, a rash, or an injury, I will follow the advice of my doctors.

Much of the skyrocketing costs of health care are the result of the medical industry treating only the symptoms of chronic health problems. Despite its treatments failing to cure chronic health problems, the medical industry is asking the government to fund its failing practices. The nation needs a change in health care strategies.

New health care leadership should …

- create more freedom to offer alternative health care services and nutritional supplements,
- encourage more alternative competition with the medical industry,
- create a new governmental agency, independent from the FDA, whose role is to promote and support wellness and alternative health care practices and fund wellness research,
- provide governmental funds for research into the relationships between symptoms and causes and the roles of cells, and
- urge health insurance suppliers to cover the costs of alternative health care products and services.

To stay in the wellness zone, I do the following:

- I try to give my body what is good for the body and not expose my body to what is bad for it.
- I try to eat most foods that are high in nutritional content and few foods that are high in calories and low in nutrition.
- I take nutritional supplements daily.

Many nutritional supplement sources are available online and over the counter. I buy from both. This book intentionally does not recommend specific sources. However, if the reader would like my opinions, they are posted on www.NaturalHealthNow.us.

Finally, I want to address the topic of sickness. This book asserts that sickness is the result of malfunctioning cells—that is, if it is not a genetic disorder. It also asserts that the cause of malfunctioning cells is typically nutritional deficiencies, and chronic nutritional deficiencies will lead to chronic health problems. If the cause is chronic nutritional deficiencies, then supplying the body with the missing nutrients should lead to properly functioning cells and a resolution of chronic health problems.

A word of advice to those who want to address their chronic health problems by taking nutritional supplements. If you are suffering from a chronic nutritional deficiency, your cells have totally depleted their inventories of one or more nutrients. Correcting malfunctioning cells will require …

- rebuilding those nutrients' inventories in each cell,
- correcting malfunctioning components of each cell, and
- creating new connective tissue to replace defective connective tissue, if connective tissue is involved.

This process takes time and will depend on how quickly cell nutritional inventories can be rebuilt and how extensive the defective components are. As a general rule, corrective action typically takes three to six months—that is, if you are supplementing with the nutrients that are missing.

Since the body only provides clues of which nutrients are missing, a more effective strategy is to take supplements that deliver a broad spectrum of nutrients. That raises the probability of providing all the nutrients the body is missing. Part of chapter 4 is devoted to developing a nutritional supplementation program.

In closing, this book reflects my concept of natural health, which is based on what we know about the body and assumptions about things we do not know about the body. I believe it is why I have no major chronic disorders at the age of eighty-three.

You are responsible for your health care. Your doctors are not responsible. Your parents are not responsible. The government is not responsible. I hope this book will help you make wise decisions.